BENEFITS OF REGULAR EXERCISE

Discussing the power of exercising regularly

Doris A. Freema

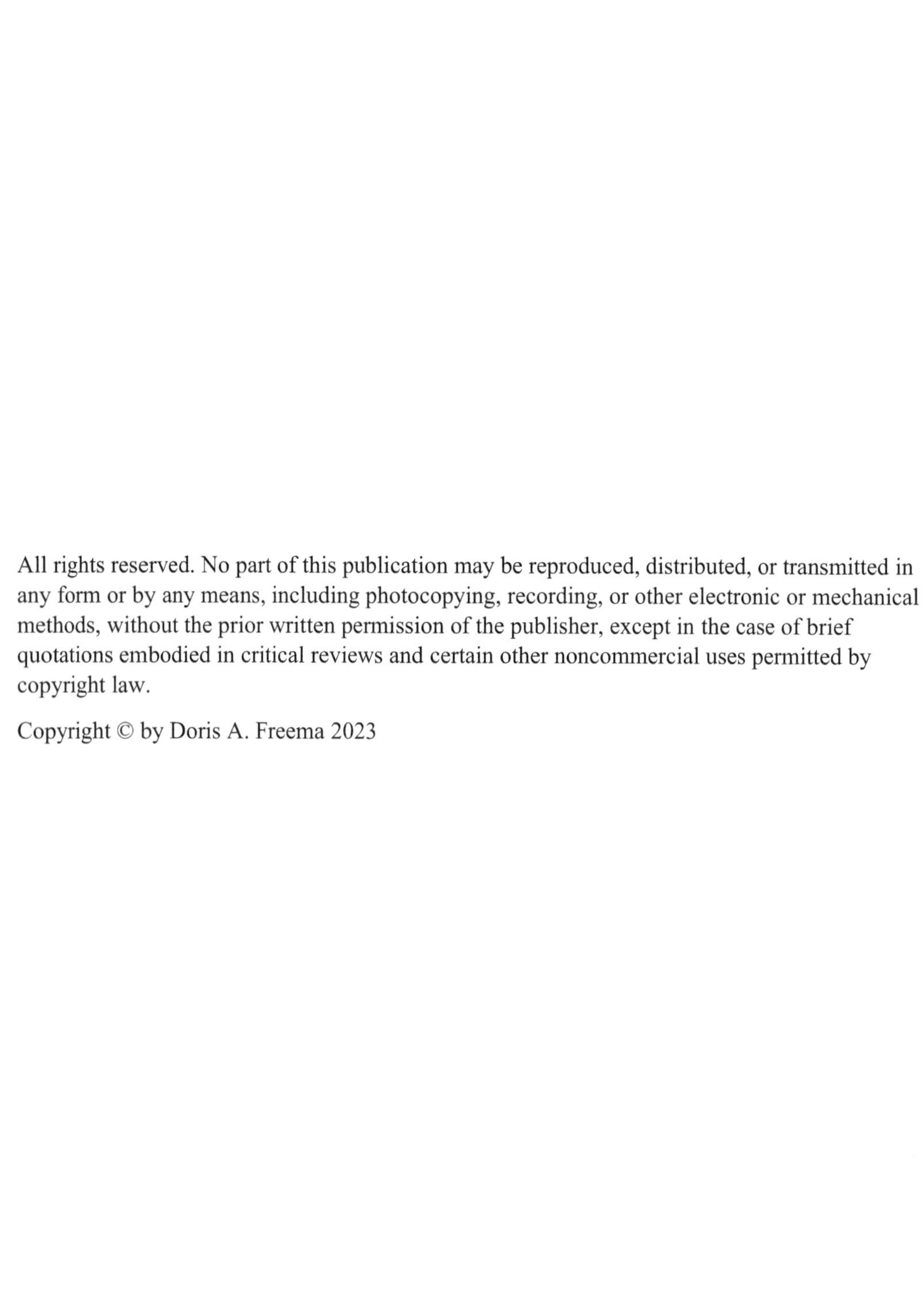

Table of content

INTRODUCTION

In today's fast-paced and sedentary lifestyle, regular exercise has become more critical than ever for maintaining good health and overall well-being. Regular exercise refers to engaging in physical activities consistently as part of a structured routine to improve and maintain physical fitness. Whether it's hitting the gym, going for a run, practicing yoga, or simply taking a brisk walk, incorporating regular exercise into our daily lives offers a lot of benefits for our body and mind.

Regular exercise is not merely about sculpting a perfect body or achieving a certain aesthetic; it goes far beyond that. It is about nurturing a healthier and more vibrant life. When we move our bodies and challenge our physical limits, we set in motion a series of positive changes that impact us at the cellular level. The definition of regular exercise varies for different individuals based on their age, fitness level, and health goals.

For some, it may involve intense workouts and weightlifting sessions, while for others, it might be gentle stretching exercises or low-impact activities. The key is consistency. Regular exercise is not a one-time event or a short-lived commitment; it is a lifelong journey toward better health. Throughout history, humans have been naturally inclined to move and engage in physical activities to survive and thrive. However, with modern conveniences and technology, physical activity has become less inherent in our daily lives.

This has led to a rise in sedentary behaviors and a decline in overall fitness levels, contributing to various health issues. In recent years, scientific research has extensively demonstrated the incredible benefits of regular exercise on our bodies and minds. Physical activity has been linked to reducing the risk of chronic diseases such as heart disease, type 2 diabetes, and certain cancers.

It helps maintain a healthy weight, improves cardiovascular health, strengthens bones and muscles, and enhances flexibility and balance. Beyond the physical advantages, regular exercise is a potent stress buster and mood enhancer. It releases endorphins, often referred to as "feel-good" hormones, which can alleviate feelings of anxiety, depression, and stress. Engaging in physical activity can boost

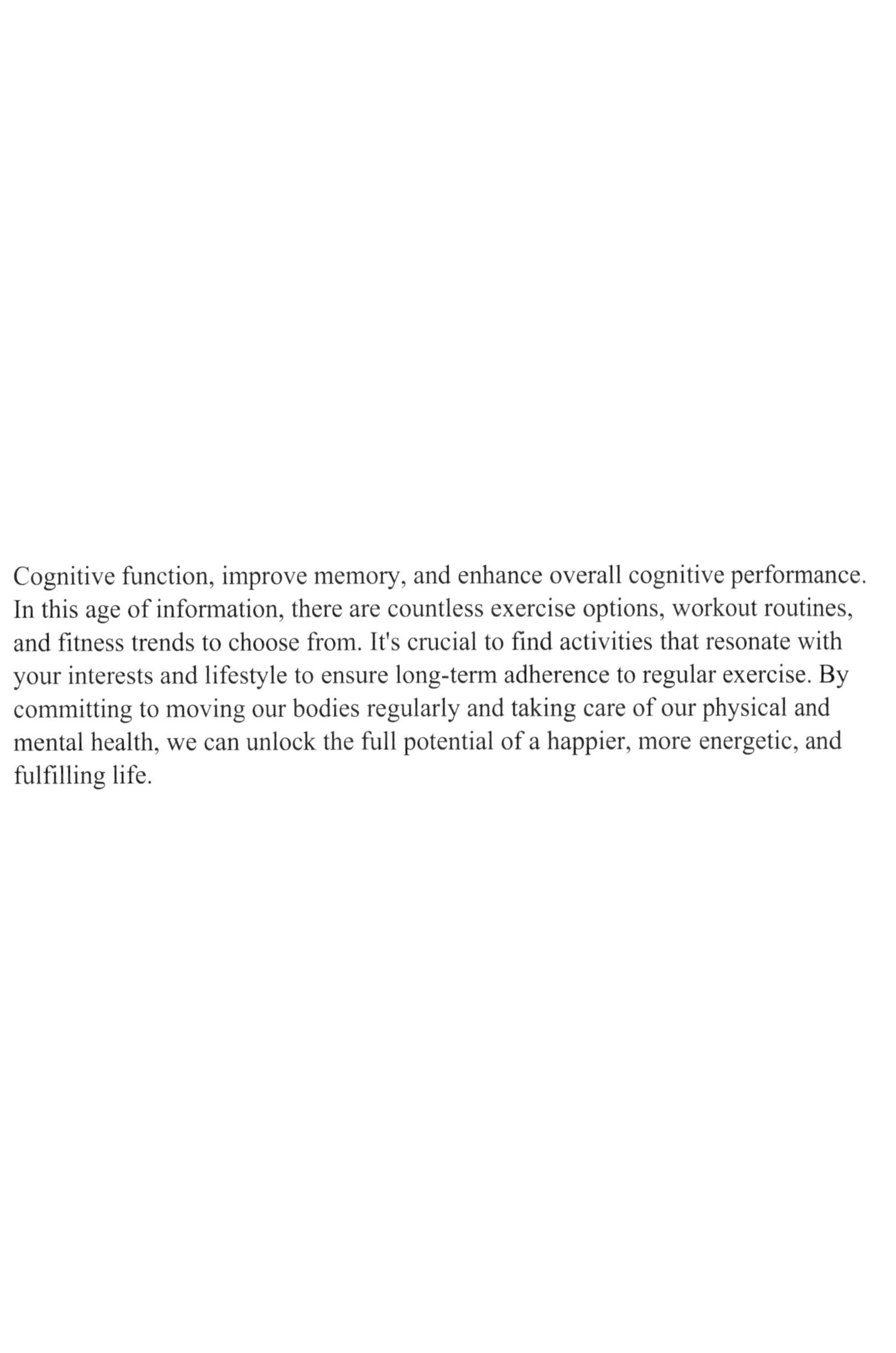

Cognitive function, improve memory, and enhance overall cognitive performance. In this age of information, there are countless exercise options, workout routines, and fitness trends to choose from. It's crucial to find activities that resonate with your interests and lifestyle to ensure long-term adherence to regular exercise. By committing to moving our bodies regularly and taking care of our physical and mental health, we can unlock the full potential of a happier, more energetic, and fulfilling life.

CHAPTER ONE

Importance of physical activity for overall health

Physical activity plays a pivotal role in achieving and maintaining overall health and well-being. Its importance extends beyond merely improving physical fitness; it positively impacts various aspects of our body, mind, and emotions. There some key reasons why physical activity is crucial for overall health.

Cardiovascular Health, Regular physical activity, such as aerobic exercises (e.g., running, swimming, cycling), strengthens the heart and improves circulation. It lowers blood pressure, reduces the risk of heart disease, and enhances cardiovascular endurance.

Weight Management: Engaging in physical activity helps burn calories and build muscle mass, contributing to weight management and preventing obesity. It also increases the body's metabolic rate, making it easier to maintain a healthy weight.

Muscle Strength and Bone Density: Resistance training and weight-bearing exercises (e.g., weight lifting, brisk walking) help build and maintain muscle mass and bone density, reducing the risk of osteoporosis and fractures, especially as we age.

Flexibility and Balance: Activities like yoga and stretching exercises promote flexibility and improve balance, reducing the likelihood of injuries and falls.

Mental Health: Physical activity is a potent mood booster. It stimulates the release of endorphins, the body's natural feel-good chemicals, which reduce stress, anxiety, and depression. Regular exercise can also improve sleep patterns and cognitive function, enhancing overall mental well-being.

Disease Prevention: Physical activity is associated with a decreased risk of several chronic conditions, including type 2 diabetes, certain cancers (e.g., colon and breast cancer), and metabolic syndrome.

Immune System Support: Regular exercise can strengthen the immune system, making the body more resilient against infections and illnesses.

Energy and Vitality: Contrary to common belief, physical activity increases energy levels. Engaging in regular exercise boosts stamina and reduces fatigue, leading to increased productivity and a greater sense of vitality.

Cognitive Function: Exercise has been linked to improved cognitive abilities, such as better memory, focus, and attention span. It may also help reduce the risk of cognitive decline and neurodegenerative diseases, like Alzheimer's.

Social Interaction: Participating in group exercises or sports provides opportunities for social interaction and fosters a sense of community, promoting mental and emotional well-being.

Longevity: Studies consistently show that individuals who engage in regular physical activity tend to live longer, healthier lives compared to those who lead sedentary lifestyles.

It's important to note that the benefits of physical activity are dose-dependent, meaning the more consistently and vigorously you engage in exercise, the greater the positive impact on your health. Incorporating physical activity into your daily routine is not only a means to improve your health but also an investment in a higher quality of life, increased longevity, and a happier, more vibrant you.

CHAPTER TWO

Weight management and prevention of obesity

Regular exercise offers a multitude of physical benefits, and one of the most prominent advantages is its role in weight management and obesity prevention. Let's delve into how consistent physical activity helps individuals maintain a healthy weight and combat obesity:

Calorie Burning: Engaging in physical activities like running, cycling, swimming, or even brisk walking burns calories. When we expend more calories through exercise than we consume through our diet, it creates a calorie deficit, leading to weight loss or weight maintenance, depending on our goals.

Muscle Building: Exercises like strength training and resistance workouts promote the development of lean muscle mass. Muscle tissue has a higher metabolic rate than fat tissue, meaning that the more muscle you have, the more calories your body burns even at rest.

Boosting Metabolism: Regular exercise revs up the body's metabolic rate, making it more efficient at processing energy from food. This increase in metabolism helps with weight management and can prevent weight gain over time.

Appetite Regulation: Physical activity can influence hormones that control appetite, leading to better appetite regulation. Some studies suggest that exercise can suppress hunger hormones and increase satiety hormones, which may result in decreased calorie intake.

Preventing Fat Accumulation: Exercise helps prevent the excessive accumulation of fat in the body by using stored fat as a source of energy during physical activity. This helps reduce overall body fat percentage and contributes to a leaner physique.

Improving Insulin Sensitivity: Regular exercise enhances insulin sensitivity, making the body's cells more responsive to insulin. This effect helps regulate blood sugar levels and reduces the risk of developing insulin resistance and type 2 diabetes, which can be associated with obesity.

Long-Term Weight Maintenance: People who engage in regular exercise are more likely to maintain their weight loss over the long term compared to those who solely rely on dieting. Exercise helps preserve muscle mass during weight loss and prevents the drop in metabolism that often accompanies calorie-restricted diets.

Healthy Fat Distribution: Some types of exercise, especially resistance training, can lead to a healthier distribution of body fat. It promotes fat loss from visceral fat (fat stored around organs) and favors subcutaneous fat (fat stored just under the skin), which is less harmful to health.

Promoting Overall Health: Obesity is a risk factor for various health conditions, including heart disease, high blood pressure, and certain cancers. By maintaining a healthy weight through regular exercise, individuals can reduce their risk of developing obesity-related health issues.

It's important to note that while exercise plays a significant role in weight management, a balanced diet and lifestyle are also crucial factors. Combining regular physical activity with a nutritious diet can optimize the benefits and support long-term weight maintenance and overall health.

Regular exercise is an effective tool for weight management and obesity prevention. By incorporating physical activity into our daily lives, we can burn calories, build lean muscle mass, boost metabolism, and improve overall health, leading to a more balanced and healthier body weight.

CHAPTER THREE

Strengthening of muscles and bones

Regular exercise provides significant benefits when it comes to strengthening muscles and bones. Whether through resistance training, weight-bearing exercises, or other forms of physical activity, consistent workouts play a pivotal role in enhancing the structural integrity and function of our musculoskeletal system. Let's explore how exercise contributes to the strengthening of muscles and bones.

Resistance Training: Activities that involve lifting weights, using resistance bands, or working with bodyweight exercises are excellent for building muscle strength. As the muscles contract against the resistance, they adapt and become stronger over time. Resistance training targets specific muscle groups, leading to increased muscle mass and improved overall strength.

Weight-Bearing Exercises: Weight-bearing activities, such as walking, running, dancing, and hiking, place stress on the bones. This stress signals the body to reinforce bone density and structure, reducing the risk of osteoporosis and fractures, especially in weight-bearing bones like the hips, spine, and legs.

Enhanced Muscle Endurance: Regular exercise not only increases muscle strength but also improves muscle endurance. Endurance exercises like cycling, swimming, or circuit training help the muscles sustain activity for longer periods without fatigue.

Joint Stability: Strengthening the muscles around the joints provides added support and stability. This is particularly beneficial for individuals with joint issues or those engaged in high-impact activities like running or sports.

Hormonal Influence: Exercise stimulates the release of growth hormones, such as testosterone and growth hormone, which aid in muscle repair and growth. Additionally, physical activity supports the release of hormones like estrogen in women, which can help maintain bone health.

Maintaining Bone Mass: As we age, there is a natural decline in bone density, leading to an increased risk of osteoporosis. Weight-bearing exercises and resistance training can help counteract this decline by preserving bone mass and reducing bone loss.

Prevention of Sarcopenia: Sarcopenia is the age-related loss of muscle mass and strength. Regular exercise, especially resistance training, can slow down this process and improve functional capacity in older adults.

Balance and Coordination: Strengthening muscles contributes to better balance and coordination, reducing the risk of falls and related injuries, especially in older adults.

Posture Improvement: Strong muscles, particularly those in the core and back, play a crucial role in maintaining good posture. Regular exercise can help alleviate issues related to poor posture.

Functional Independence: Strengthened muscles and bones are essential for performing daily activities with ease and maintaining functional independence throughout life.

It's important to engage in a variety of exercises that target different muscle groups and include both weight-bearing and resistance exercises. Additionally, progressive overload (gradually increasing the intensity or resistance of exercises) is essential to continue challenging muscles and bones for continued growth and adaptation.

 Regular exercise, particularly through resistance training and weight-bearing activities, plays a key role in strengthening muscles and bones. These physical adaptations not only enhance functional capacity but also promote overall health, mobility, and independence, making exercise a vital component of a healthy lifestyle.

CHAPTER FOUR

Reduction of the risk of chronic diseases such as heart disease and type 2 diabetes

Reducing the risk of chronic diseases such as heart disease and type 2 diabetes is crucial for maintaining overall health and well-being. Several lifestyle factors play a significant role in minimizing the risk of these diseases.

Balanced Diet: Adopting a healthy and balanced diet is vital in preventing chronic diseases. Limit the intake of processed foods, sugary beverages, and excessive amounts of salt.

Regular Exercise: Engaging in regular physical activity has numerous health benefits, including reducing the risk of heart disease and type 2 diabetes.

Weight Management: Maintaining a healthy weight or achieving weight loss if necessary can significantly reduce the risk of chronic diseases. Excess body weight, especially around the abdomen, is associated with an increased risk of heart disease and type 2 diabetes.

Avoiding Tobacco and Limiting Alcohol: Smoking is a major risk factor for heart disease and other chronic illnesses, including cancer. Quitting smoking is one of the best things you can do for your health. Additionally, excessive alcohol consumption can lead to various health issues, so it's essential to drink in moderation or avoid alcohol altogether.

Stress Management: Chronic stress can contribute to the development of chronic diseases. Finding healthy ways to manage stress, such as practicing mindfulness, meditation, or engaging in hobbies, can be beneficial.

Regular Health Checkups: Regular health checkups can help identify risk factors and early signs of chronic diseases. Regular visits to your healthcare provider can lead to early detection and appropriate management.

Sleep: getting enough sleep each night. Poor sleep patterns have been linked to an increased risk of chronic diseases.

Blood Pressure and Cholesterol Management: Monitoring and managing blood pressure and cholesterol levels are crucial for preventing heart disease. High blood pressure and high cholesterol are significant risk factors for cardiovascular issues.

Diabetes Prevention: For type 2 diabetes prevention, maintaining a healthy lifestyle, including a balanced diet and regular exercise, is crucial. For individuals at high risk, regular blood sugar screenings may be necessary. Community Support: Engaging with supportive social networks and communities can encourage healthy behaviors and help maintain a healthier lifestyle.

Remember, individual factors, such as genetics and family history, can also influence the risk of chronic diseases. While we cannot control these factors, adopting a healthy lifestyle can significantly improve overall health and reduce the risk of developing heart disease, type 2 diabetes, and other chronic conditions. Always consult a healthcare professional for personalized advice and guidance.

CHAPTER FIVE

Improvement in mood and reduction of stress and anxiety

Regular exercise offers a multitude of mental and cognitive benefits, and indeed, improvement in mood and reduction of stress and anxiety are among the most prominent ones. Here's a closer look at how exercise positively impacts mental health and cognitive functioning:

Mood: Regular exercise improves and stimulates the release of endorphins, which are called feel-good elevators. This natural chemicals promote a sense of happiness and well-being, leading to an improved mood.

Stress Reduction: Engaging in physical activity can reduce the body's stress hormones, such as cortisol. It acts as a natural stress reliever, helping to lower tension and enhance the ability to cope with stressful situations.

Anxiety Reduction: Exercise can reduce symptoms of anxiety and help manage generalized anxiety disorder. It provides a distraction from anxious thoughts, releases tension, and promotes relaxation.

Cognitive Function: Regular exercise enhanced cognitive function, which includes attention better memory, and problem-solving skills. Physical activity increases blood flow to the brain, promoting the growth of new neurons and enhancing brain plasticity.

Boosted Brain Health: Exercise is associated with a reduced risk of cognitive decline and neurodegenerative diseases, such as Alzheimer's disease. It may help maintain brain health and cognitive abilities as we age.

Increased Focus and Concentration: Physical activity has been shown to enhance focus and concentration, which can improve productivity and overall cognitive performance.

Better Sleep: Regular exercise can contribute to better sleep quality and can help alleviate insomnia. Improved sleep, in turn, positively affects mental and emotional well-being.

Enhanced Self-Esteem and Body Image: Regular exercise can lead to improvements in body image and self-esteem, especially when individuals achieve their fitness goals or notice positive changes in their bodies.

Social Interaction and Support: Participating in group exercises or sports can provide social interaction and support, which can have positive effects on mental well-being.

Mind-Body Connection: Certain exercises, such as yoga and tai chi, emphasize the mind-body connection, promoting mindfulness and relaxation.

It's important to note that while exercise can be beneficial for mental health, it is not a substitute for professional treatment in cases of severe depression, anxiety disorders, or other mental health conditions.

If you or someone you know is struggling with mental health issues, it's essential to seek help from a qualified mental health professional.

Regular exercise not only improves physical health but also has a profound impact on mental and cognitive well-being. Incorporating physical activity into daily life can lead to a happier, less stressed, and more focused and resilient mind.

CHAPTER SIX

Boost in self-confidence and self esteem

Regular exercise can lead to a boost in self-confidence and self-esteem in several ways:

Achievement and Progress: Setting and achieving fitness goals can give a sense of accomplishment and pride. As individuals progress in their exercise routines, they can see tangible improvements in their strength, endurance, flexibility, and overall fitness. This sense of progress can boost self-confidence and motivate individuals to continue their fitness journey.

Body Image: Exercise can lead to positive changes in body composition and overall physical appearance. Engaging in regular physical activity can help individuals feel more comfortable and confident in their bodies, improving body image and self-perception.

Stress Reduction: As mentioned earlier, exercise is an excellent stress reliever. When stress is managed effectively, it can positively impact self-esteem and self-confidence, as individuals feel more in control of their emotions and responses to challenging situations.

Neurotransmitters and Hormones: Exercise stimulates the release of endorphins, dopamine, and serotonin, which are neurotransmitters associated with feelings of happiness, pleasure, and overall well-being. These neurochemicals play a significant role in boosting mood and enhancing self-esteem.

Social Interaction: Participating in group exercise classes, team sports, or fitness communities can provide social interaction and a sense of belonging. Positive interactions and support from others can contribute to increased self-esteem and confidence.

Empowerment: Regular exercise empowers individuals by demonstrating their ability to take charge of their health and well-being. The knowledge that they are actively working towards improving themselves can significantly boost self-confidence.

Coping Skills: Regular exercise can serve as a healthy coping mechanism for dealing with life's challenges. Instead of turning to negative coping strategies, individuals may find empowerment in using exercise as a positive outlet. Cognitive Benefits: Improved cognitive function resulting from regular exercise can lead to enhanced problem-solving skills and decision-making abilities. This, in turn, can contribute to a sense of self-assurance in various aspects of life.

Body Positivity: Engaging in physical activity can foster a more positive and accepting attitude towards one's body, emphasizing its strength, resilience, and capabilities rather than solely focusing on appearance. Emphasizing Self-Care: Prioritizing exercise as a form of self-care sends a powerful message of self-worth and self-respect. Taking time for oneself and engaging in activities that promote well-being can significantly impact self-esteem.

The benefits of exercise on self-esteem and self-confidence may vary from person to person. Additionally, it's essential to approach exercise with a healthy and balanced perspective, avoiding excessive self-criticism or unrealistic expectations. The key is to find physical activities that you enjoy and that make you feel good about yourself, rather than viewing exercise as a punishment or means to achieve an idealized body image. Embrace the journey of self-improvement and celebrate the progress you make along the way.

CHAPTER SEVEN

Enhancement of cognitive functions such as memory and attention

Regular exercise has been associated with significant enhancements in cognitive functions, particularly in memory and attention. This is how exercise positively impacts these cognitive abilities:

Blood Flow to the Brain: exercise increases blood flow to the brain, supplying more oxygen and nutrients. This enhanced blood flow promotes the growth of new blood vessels and neurons, which can improve overall brain health and cognitive function.

Neurotransmitter Release: Exercise stimulates the release of various neurotransmitters, such as dopamine and norepinephrine. These chemicals play essential roles in regulating attention and focus, leading to improved concentration and mental alertness.

Brain-Derived Neurotrophic Factor (BDNF): Exercise promotes the release of BDNF, a protein that supports the growth and maintenance of brain cells. BDNF plays a vital role in synaptic plasticity, the process by which neurons form and strengthen connections, contributing to enhanced memory and learning abilities.

Hippocampus Growth: The hippocampus, a region of the brain critical for memory formation and storage, can experience increased volume through regular exercise. This structural change has been linked to improved memory function.

Stress Reduction: As mentioned earlier, exercise is an effective stress reducer. Lowering stress levels can enhance cognitive functions, as chronic stress can impair memory and attention.

Improved Sleep Quality: Regular exercise can lead to better sleep quality, which is essential for memory consolidation and cognitive performance.

Cognitive Reserve: Engaging in physical activity throughout life is associated with a concept known as cognitive reserve. This refers to the brain's ability to resist damage and maintain cognitive function despite age-related changes or neurological insults.

Executive Function: Exercise has shown positive effects on executive functions, which involve higher-order cognitive processes such as problem-solving, planning, and decision-making.

Neuroplasticity: Exercise can increase neuroplasticity, which is the brain's ability to reorganize and form new neural connections. This adaptability is crucial for learning and memory processes.

Mental Stimulation: Certain types of exercise, such as activities that require coordination and skill, can provide mental stimulation, challenging the brain and supporting cognitive functions.

It's important to note that while exercise can enhance cognitive functions, it is not a standalone solution. Leading a healthy lifestyle that includes a balanced diet, adequate sleep, and mental engagement is essential for maintaining cognitive health. Additionally, individual responses to exercise may vary, and the benefits might be more pronounced in some individuals than others.

To maximize the cognitive benefits of exercise, it's advisable to engage in a variety of physical activities, including aerobic exercises (e.g., brisk walking, jogging, cycling) and activities that involve coordination and balance (e.g., dancing, yoga). Aim for regular exercise sessions, as consistency is key in reaping the cognitive rewards of physical activity.

CHAPTER EIGHT

Opportunities for social interaction and making new friends

Engaging in regular exercise not only offers numerous physical health benefits but also provides valuable opportunities for social interaction and the chance to make new friends. Here are some of the social benefits of participating in exercise activities that foster social interaction:

Community Building: Exercise classes, sports teams, and group activities create a sense of belonging and community. People with shared interests in fitness and health often form strong bonds, leading to a supportive social network.

New Friendships: Participating in group exercises, sports leagues, or fitness clubs can lead to meeting people who share similar interests. This can lead to the formation of new friendships, providing individuals with social connections that enrich their lives.

Increased Social Engagement: Regular exercise often involves interacting with others during the activity, before and after sessions, and during breaks. These interactions encourage conversation and social engagement, fostering connections beyond the exercise itself.

Motivation and Accountability: Exercising with friends or in a group setting can enhance motivation and accountability. People are more likely to stick to their exercise routines when they have others counting on them or when they enjoy the company of their workout partners.

Reduced Isolation: Engaging in exercise-related social activities can help combat feelings of loneliness and isolation. Regular interactions with others contribute to a sense of belonging and emotional well-being.

Diverse Social Circles: Exercise environments often bring together individuals from diverse backgrounds, promoting interactions with people who might not be part of one's usual social circles. This exposure can lead to increased understanding and cultural awareness.

Shared Goals and Achievements: Working towards fitness goals as a group can create a sense of camaraderie. Celebrating shared achievements, whether completing a challenging workout or reaching personal milestones, strengthens social bonds.

Stress Reduction: Socializing during exercise can help reduce stress and anxiety. Engaging in physical activities with others can serve as a distraction from daily worries and provide an outlet for relaxation.

Skill Sharing and Learning: Group exercise activities offer opportunities for skill sharing and learning. More experienced participants often help newcomers, fostering a sense of mentorship and mutual support.

Positive Peer Pressure: Surrounding oneself with like-minded individuals who prioritize health and fitness can lead to positive peer pressure. This can motivate individuals to maintain healthy habits and make positive lifestyle choices.

Improved Mental Health: Social interactions and connections fostered through exercise have been shown to contribute to improved mental health outcomes, including reduced symptoms of depression and anxiety.

 Overall, participating in exercise activities that encourage social interaction and the opportunity to make new friends can have a profound impact on an individual's well-being. These interactions not only enhance physical health but also contribute to emotional and social wellness.

CHAPTER NINE

Promotion of teamwork and cooperation through group activities or sports

Participating in group activities or sports is an excellent way to promote teamwork, cooperation, and valuable interpersonal skills.

Shared Goals: Group activities and sports require participants to work towards a common goal. Whether it's winning a game, completing a challenge, or achieving a collective objective, individuals learn to align their efforts and skills to accomplish something together.

Communication: Effective communication is crucial in group activities and sports. Players need to convey their intentions, share information, and coordinate strategies to achieve success. Clear communication promotes understanding and minimizes misunderstandings.

Collaboration: Participants in group activities learn to collaborate by combining their strengths and compensating for weaknesses. This collaborative effort ensures that everyone contributes to the team's overall performance.

Problem-Solving: Challenges and obstacles are common in group activities and sports. Working together to solve problems cultivates critical thinking and creative problem-solving skills. Participants learn to adapt, adjust strategies, and make quick decisions under pressure.

Trust Building: Successful teamwork relies on trust. Through consistent interactions, individuals develop trust in their teammate's abilities, judgment, and commitment. This trust leads to a sense of reliability and mutual support.

Role Definition: Team sports often require individuals to play specific roles based on their strengths and skills. This encourages participants to understand their unique contributions and how they fit into the larger team structure.

Empathy and Understanding: Engaging with diverse teammates allows individuals to learn about different perspectives, backgrounds, and experiences. This fosters empathy and understanding, promoting a more inclusive and harmonious team environment.

Dispute Resolution: Disputes are unavoidable in any partnership environment. Through group activities and sports, participants develop skills in resolving conflicts constructively, understanding compromise, and maintaining positive relationships.

Motivation and Accountability: Teammates hold each other accountable for their performance and commitment. The desire to contribute and not let others down serves as motivation to stay engaged and give their best effort.

Leadership Development: Within a team, leaders naturally emerge. Group activities provide opportunities for individuals to take on leadership roles, guiding and motivating others. This helps in nurturing leadership qualities and skills.

Sportsmanship: Group activities and sports emphasize the importance of fair play, respect for opponents, and graceful acceptance of both victories and defeats. These values contribute to the development of good sportsmanship.

Social Bonds: Engaging in group activities and sports encourages the formation of strong social bonds. These connections extend beyond the activity itself, fostering friendships and support networks.

Learning to Win and Lose Gracefully: Experiencing wins and losses as a team teaches participants how to handle success with humility and failure with resilience. These lessons are valuable in various aspects of life.

CHAPTER TEN

Improvement in overall quality of life and happiness levels

Engaging in regular physical activity, whether through sports, exercise, or group activities, has been linked to significant improvements in overall quality of life and happiness levels.

Physical Health Benefits: Regular exercise and physical activity are associated with improved physical health, including better cardiovascular health, stronger muscles and bones, and a reduced risk of chronic diseases such as diabetes and obesity. When your body feels healthier, it positively impacts your overall well-being and happiness.

Mental Health: Exercise is known to release endorphins, which are often referred to as "feel-good" hormones. These endorphins can help alleviate feelings of stress, anxiety, and depression, contributing to better mental health and an increased sense of happiness.

Stress Reduction: Engaging in physical activities can serve as a form of stress relief. Physical exertion helps release tension and provides an outlet for built-up stress, promoting a sense of relaxation and well-being.

Improved Mood: Exercise has been shown to boost mood by increasing the levels of neurotransmitters like serotonin and dopamine. This can lead to feelings of happiness, contentment, and reduced mood swings.

Increased Energy Levels: Regular physical activity can increase your overall energy levels, making you feel more alert, focused, and motivated. This improved energy contributes to a greater sense of vitality and satisfaction in daily life.

Enhanced Self-Esteem: Achieving fitness goals, participating in group activities, and experiencing personal growth through physical challenges can boost self-

Esteem and self-confidence. Feeling accomplished in these areas translates into a more positive self-perception and increased happiness.

Social Interaction: Participating in group activities or sports provides opportunities for social interaction and the formation of meaningful connections. These social bonds contribute to a sense of belonging and happiness.

Cognitive Benefits: Physical activity has been linked to improved cognitive function, including better memory, focus, and problem-solving skills. This can lead to a greater sense of accomplishment and cognitive well-being.

Mind-Body Connection: Engaging in activities that require coordination and physical effort can enhance the mind-body connection. This connection is associated with a greater sense of mindfulness and an increased appreciation for the present moment.

Quality Sleep: Regular exercise can help regulate sleep patterns, leading to better sleep quality. Adequate sleep is essential for overall well-being and can significantly impact your mood and happiness levels.

Sense of Achievement: Setting and achieving fitness goals, whether small or significant, can provide a sense of accomplishment. This feeling of progress and growth contributes to higher overall life satisfaction.

Positive Lifestyle Habits: Engaging in physical activities often leads to adopting healthier lifestyle habits, such as improved nutrition and reduced sedentary behavior. These positive changes can have a cascading effect on overall well-being and happiness.

Personal Fulfillment: Engaging in activities that challenge you physically and mentally can lead to a sense of personal fulfillment and a deeper appreciation for your capabilities.

Overall, the combination of physical, mental, emotional, and social benefits derived from regular physical activity and participation in group activities can lead to an improved overall quality of life and elevated levels of happiness. It's important to find activities that you enjoy and that align with your interests and capabilities to maximize these positive effects.